ATTRACT THE MAIN GIRL; Proven Steps To Make Her Chase You

Jean R. Lesh

Table of content

Introduction

Many guys still have trouble learning how to attract women's attention or even how to find a relationship. Even for males who are already adept at seducing women, it might be challenging to locate the woman of their dreams, win her heart, and develop a strong bond with her. But it gets worse if that pressure wasn't enough. The results of his decisions will be BRUTAL if a man FAILS to discover the RIGHT woman to have a satisfying, conflict-free, and passionate relationship. A life of unfulfilling, lifeless relationships with shallow, low-character, dull, incompatible, and uninteresting women is the fate of guys who don't know how to acquire the female they REALLY want.

Chapter 1

How Relationships are Affected by Masculine and Female Energies

A more passionate relationship can result from embracing the balance of the masculine and feminine in both ourselves and our partner.

What makes two people fall in love and be attracted to one another?

Many relationship experts, including Tony Robbins and Esther Perel, investigate how the polarity of the feminine and masculine energies between two people leads to physical passion in a relationship. The stronger the attraction, the more those two energies are at odds.

Understanding how these two energies interact can help relationships develop attraction and maintain their passion.

- Understanding Polarity: Male and Female While our shared interests bind us together, the polarity of two individuals—the contrast between their masculine and feminine energies—ignites our passion. This polarity refers to the strong physical attraction that exists between two people; the more opposed the energies, the more compelling the attraction. But first, what do the masculine and feminine versions mean? In general, masculine energy pushes toward a mission and seeks to understand and resolve a problem. Feminine energy, on the other hand, values connection and seeks to connect with a partner through problem-sharing. Making Sense of Our Core Energy. In actuality, both masculine and feminine energies are present in each of us. People often have either a stronger feminine or male energy, though we can have a mix of both. However, life events like our fear of falling short or not being loved can have a significant impact on us and cause us to use "masks" to hide our true selves. Let's imagine, for illustration, that a girl is born with naturally powerful feminine energy. To prevent her from being overly reliant on a man, her mother teaches her how to construct a male mask as she grows up. She feels stronger because of her father's domineering behavior, which furthers the masculine façade. She no longer understands the natural harmony between the feminine and masculine energies since she is a woman. This hinders her from being herself and from being her true self in front of her spouse. restoring equilibrium Over time, a lot of relationships lose their intensity. When there is no longer a balance of masculine and feminine energy between partners, this happens. The polarity between two people may be abruptly destroyed if someone with feminine energy criticizes a masculine person's struggle with their life's path. A feminine individual, on the other hand, could become withdrawn and less lively when reprimanded for being fatigued. "Never tell a lady with a feminine sexual essence that she is ugly," advises David Deida. "Never tell a guy with a masculine sexual essence that he is incorrect." Developing both your masculine and feminine traits will help you rediscover your passion. If you're in a relationship, this can help you rekindle the passion and playfulness, or if you're single, it can help you meet someone interesting. You may embrace your partner's authenticity while still being yourself when you are aware of this lovely balance

2 What Women Look For in men

Most men probably do not
expect what women desire in a man. Women look for qualities in a man that genuinely define his worth.

1. honesty

Women like openness and honesty in a man more than any other quality. Being honest is a show of security, which is the point. Everything is how it appears, and nothing is being held back. It's time for men to quit acting fake and start being authentic. Honest about your abilities, flaws, and challenges. Be honest about your worries, aspirations, and hopes. Realize who you are, not who you wish you were. A woman might feel safe hiding her heart with a man who has nothing to conceal. That is macho.

2. Compassion: A guy's heart will always reveal whether he is a real man. Does he feel the same emotions that God feels? Is the suffering in his life breaking him? Is he affected by the sins he's attempting to purge? Is he impacted when circumstances, relationships, or aspects of daily life are not as they should be? A true

guy lets his emotions affect him and then lets those feelings guide his actions. a man who seeks repair, healing, and closure. a man who works hard to make things right both outside of him and inside of him. Because therein we will always discover the heart of Jesus, we are looking for guys who are kind, compassionate, and loving. The capacity to humble oneself is what elevates a man beyond all other things in the world. A genuine guy doesn't need to promote himself since his life already accomplishes that. Because a humble man is so much more concerned with his walk than his discourse, he can set aside the talk. He has set up his "rights" in favor of the freedom to be unselfish, caring, and full of grace. As a result, he is fast to listen, slow to talk, and slow to become angry. The manliest man, Jesus, is the best example of humility since he gave up his privileges and began to show his beloved spouse his unwavering love and devotion. The same is what real guys aim towards. Nothing is more desirable than a guy who emanates power.

3. Strength, but not the sort that makes your muscles tear; mental, emotional, and spiritual strength. a man's strength that stems from his ability to speak up strongly for what is right. a quality of being able to distinguish between right and wrong and admit when they have been crossed. a quality of being self-assured enough to act morally and make wise decisions. Women want men who can stand on their own in this day of compromise, standing on to their values, beliefs, and most importantly, their principles.

4. Purity: Our culture has deceived us into believing that males cannot control their eyes and that women cannot control their

emotions. This is a falsehood right out of the bowels of hell, in my opinion. Interacting with women who assume their husbands would succumb to desire, infidelity, and adultery as if it were inevitable makes me feel sick. our world is certainly filled with sexual temptation and challenges, but it is also true that we serve a God who grants us control over every aspect of our existence, including our minds, emotions, and bodies. When a guy has enough respect and integrity for the women in his life to refuse temptations, he is being masculine. Ladies, I don't know about you, but I enabled a guy precisely like him to capture my heart. He is a guy who seeks to maintain honesty, integrity, strength, compassion, and humility in his life and our relationship, even though I can state with confidence that he is far from perfect. Now is the moment to demand more from our guys and then patiently wait till you see these traits in action in his life. Do not compromise for anything less. when circumstances, relationships, or aspects of daily life are not as they should be? A true guy lets his emotions affect him and then lets those feelings guide his actions

Chapter 2

Create a powerful male figure to surround her with

It is good to have the drive to advance both your relationship and oneself. This wish is not shared by many others. The male energy is the cup that holds and sustains the feminine energy if you see it as water (free, flowing, and unfettered). Take meaningful acts to surprise your girlfriend while being affectionate and caring. She could want you to defend her more, or to look out for her more; she might want you to get more exercise, or to make more male friends.

1. Show greater sincerity. Being true to yourself is the greatest approach to being

more manly in a relationship. Being able to look for oneself helps you to be more real. You have a strong desire to grow, learn, take on responsibility, and honor your commitments. You appreciate others and are prepared to look out for and take care of those who are less strong or capable of taking care of themselves. You don't want attention and are modest. If people want to take care of themselves, you're ready to stand aside and let them. Accepting a man's genuine nature and his desire to fit in with himself, his family, and society are two characteristics of authentic masculinity. Authenticity simply refers to being true to who you are despite external pressure to change you or what you are. You are honest with yourself, your relationship, and other people, and you take ownership of your errors. Your deeds, ideas, and principles all line- up.

Treat her like a queen by walking on her right side, opening doors for her, cuddling up to her on the sofa, and walking the dog. An equal relationship is impossible; a dominant part of the relationship is necessary. Typically, the woman is unhappy with having to be the dominant part. You will be able to do it because of this.

2. Pay closer attention. If your partner has a feminine core, draw attention to them, reassure them, and show them that you understand them. Instead of making them feel invisible, unsafe, or misunderstood, make them feel seen, safe, and understood. The masculine energy is the cup that holds and supports the feminine energy if you picture it as water (free, flowing, and unrestricted) Take heartfelt actions to surprise your girlfriend while being loving and caring. She might want you to defend

her more, or to look out for her more; she might want you to get more exercise, or to make more male friends.

3. Show more confidence. Make your own choices and follow your direction, frequently defying the influence of others, including your girlfriend. However, this does not negate the need for a dictatorship. Develop the ability to act decisively and assume control when necessary without using excessive force or aggression. When the Masculine takes the initiative, the Feminine can relax in confidence and respect how much thought you put into any decisions, which is a quality the Feminine values in a partner. She wants to know that you can defend her from danger and that your admiration for her beauty has made you decide against seeking out a new partner.

Chapter 3

selecting the ideal girlfriend

We'll get into the first subject in this essay. You'll save a lot of time, heartache, and hassle if you can learn how to pick your girlfriend. There isn't a perfect girl, and this article isn't intended to encourage you to start looking for someone who doesn't exist. Even if you do manage to locate a virgin or female who has only slept with one guy, who is feminine, youthful, and seems to be the perfect match, you can always end the relationship by contracting oneitis and having her cheat on you or dump you. The likelihood that your relationship will continue for a long time will significantly rise if you know how to choose your partner. Additionally, it will vastly improve the standard of the connection and your experience in it.

There are benefits to having a girlfriend, regardless of whether you're simply sick of being a player, want company while you grow your career, want to have a family, or are just curious about what a relationship may provide you. Even the most dominant male can take the lead in any relationship, but it will be a lot simpler if you locate a good female first, and then lead correctly from there.

How can I find a good girlfriend?

So how do you decide which female to choose?

Finding a female with a positive general is the first step in the process. You can always screw up by elevating the pussy, or you can try the difficult route of trying to turn a hoe into a housewife. But it's simply so much simpler when you discover a lady who already has good attributes. You must decide on the traits you want in a partner. Some of the work has been done for you by myself.

Characteristics of a superior girlfriend

1. Low notch count: lying in bed and getting your ex back. If you're learning how to choose a girlfriend, you should look for a female with a modest notch count. In other words, she has slept with the fewest men conceivable. Though improbable, a virgin is always desirable. I set a strict cutoff at 12, but in reality, you want a female with a notch count of no more than five. Better off with less than.

There is nothing wrong with women who hold higher-ranking positions. In actuality, I get along well with seasoned ladies. And the majority of the ladies you fuck will have 20 to 30 or more notch counts. There are many gorgeous, seductive ladies with notch counts of 20, 25, or even 30 fellas. However, you cannot become their girlfriend. least of all intentionally. It's not entirely your responsibility if she flat-out lies to you about how many notches she has. However, you should be aware that while deciding how to choose your partner, ladies with high notch counts are far from ideal. She finds it simpler to let go of sex and move to the more guys she has slept with. This implies that if things aren't going well in the relationship, she'll be more motivated to look for better possibilities than you.

1. Probabilities: Don't stray from the norm Undoubtedly, both high-class and low-class countess can be faithful. But it's all about probabilities when you're learning how to pick your girlfriend. And compared to a girl with a high-notch count, you're much more likely to get along well with someone who has a lower-notch count. In essence, women with higher notch counts have more games. They have improved man-handling skills and understand how to use their pussy to gain an advantage in both their relationships and the wider world. When you two start dating, this will lead to more issues. Getting a girlfriend with a lower-notch count is much preferable. No way to be certain All things considered, there is

no surefire way to determine a woman's actual notch count. You'll need to hazard a guess. One of the reasons you don't declare a girl to be your girlfriend after a few weeks or a month is due to this. For at least three to six months, you should be seeing her. In this manner, you can discover her true character. Any girl can put on a nice, sweet act for a month or even two. But you might start to glimpse a girl's actual nature after 3 or 4 months of dating her. You may learn a lot about a woman's genuine notch count by observing how she behaves, speaks, treats you, and shares her life. And often, a lady will just tell you about it or bring it up on her own. She'll ask you eventually whether she thinks highly of you. If you ask her, you'll come across as frail and feminine. So refrain from requesting her phone number. Because doing so will result in a bogus number. Let her discuss former lovers. Make her give you her number first if she's eager to get your number, as most women will be. Never respond to a question; just deflect it. I usually try to avoid questions about my notch count and never provide a straight response. When I have, I have downplayed my stature. Giving a figure between 20 and 30 is a good bet. If you have a notch count of that or above as a player, that is. You are lying if you claim to be a virgin or have a notch count of 5. However, it will be simpler to pull off underplaying it if you've slept with 50 or 60 people. An unhappy lady could have a low-notch count. However, it doesn't amount to several hundred to enough disgust or frighten her away. You look sexually experienced enough to not be a desperate beta guy, thus a lady with a notch count equal to or even greater than yours will feel confident to tell you her genuine number. A female could easily tell you 5 if you tell her your number is 3 and her true number is 25. I had her say the number first because of this. And you could even discover that a few weeks after she answers 5, and you respond with 25, she will respond with a different response. She doesn't regret lying about her number and believes she can be honest with a higher-tier count man, not because she fucked 10 men in a matter of weeks. In conclusion, it is impossible to fully determine a woman's notch count. Furthermore, you shouldn't mention it initially. Must guess and make an effort to obtain a sense of what it is. Ask yourself inquiries about her. Does she frequent parties? Or does she choose to stay home and read? Does she get along well with her parents, or did her father abandon the family when she was a child? Do her ex-boyfriends look like lovely individuals, or are they part of a gang? This is a major issue. It's a positive indicator if a female, particularly one who is between the ages of 18 and 25, spends most of her time with beta males. It indicates that she chose to try and make a relationship with a beta-type man work rather than pursuing an alpha dick at her peak years of beauty. Consequently, she values relationships more than she values just exploiting her attractiveness till she runs out of options. This leads us to our next point.

2. Red pill: *values relationships * Pursuing a connection with a person who appreciates relationships is necessary if you want to learn how to acquire a good girlfriend. Every lady in the world will tell you how important relationships are to them. That is something that even a prostitute or the local slut would say. But while pursuing a high-caliber woman, pay attention to her behavior rather than her words. You must investigate her history. For women, notch count is crucial because of this. A low-notch count, however,

only tells half of the tale. A female with an 8-notch count who is 30 years old is considerably different from a girl with the same notch count who is 18 years old. Of course, you'd choose the younger woman. But an 18-year-old girl who has dated 8 men is probably not going to value relationships the same way her elder counterpart does. For western standards, it's fairly nice if a female has dated a few guys but they have all been boyfriends, with maybe one or two one-night encounters. She may not regard relationships the same way if she has only had one boyfriend and then 8–9 one-night stands or casual sex partners.

She may desire a boyfriend, but she is open to dating men outside of that group.

And while I enjoy women who engage in extramarital sex, I also enjoy spending time with them in that exact context. not in a romantic relationship.

Relationship-oriented girls, It's important to be able to tell the difference between girls who genuinely value relationships and those who only do so when it's convenient if you want to know how to pick your girlfriend. The women who value relationships are the ones who are in them the majority of the time. Concerning whether or not girls are serial monogamous versus girls who remain single for a long time, there has been some discussion and inquiries I've received. Let me tell you, being with a girl who practices serial monogamy is ten times better. Only a few of them are important because the main thing is to make sure that these relationships were lasting. The girl could as well be casual if she dates a man for three months, then switches him out every three months. Go ahead from here. Long-term single women are not something I have anything against. If she is, it is likely because she is riding the cock carousel or is unable to convince a man to settle down. In either case, she's taking extra liberties, accruing debt, and making it more difficult to start new relationships. A girl who has only been in one to three relationships before yours and hasn't done much else is committed to making a relationship work. In the end, you want a female who is actively seeking a relationship. She's going to miss that lifestyle if you choose a girlfriend who genuinely loves her but is typically single. And very soon after you argue or split up, she'll either start cheating on you or start sucking and fucking other men. A relationship that is feminine and follows your lead guy Women can value relationships while maintaining constant control. You need a girl who is feminine and readily follows your instructions in addition to a woman who prefers relationships. The women who are most attracted to you are those that treat you with femininity and follow your example right away. Because of this, some women will behave more feminine around stronger men while acting more masculine near more beautiful or stronger males. If you start behaving beta or weak in the relationship, this might alter with time. However, if you maintain your manly attributes, you may continue to be the relationship's head. But at the moment, our attention is on how to choose a girlfriend. And certain females will be considerably more feminine than others that you'll sleep with and casually meet. recognizing a girl's femininity It will depend on both how naturally feminine she is and how much she loves you. It will be clear when a girl is feminine in any case. She'll go along with your ideas, suck your dick without your permission, want to hang out, dress femininely, and won't shit test you often. Compared to other ladies who are less submissive around you, a lady who is feminine and follows your lead from the beginning would be a far better girlfriend. A female is often at her finest when she isn't your girlfriend yet. Therefore, if she isn't being feminine right now, not much will change until you turn into the Rock. You can always keep her submissive to you and even increase throughout the relationship. But it must be there from the start. Avoid settling for the sexiest woman you can get into bed with while looking for a good partner. In contrast to the 8 or 8.5, the 9 or 10 who was eager to fuck you could like you but not be as subservient. It's preferable to start with learning how to choose your partner depending on how she makes you feel. She may, of course, be attractive as well. How to approach this girl acquiring a girlfriend and maintaining the relationship Ironically, if you date numerous women, you'll be with ladies who aren't suitable for becoming your girlfriend. Due to this, many males get jaded and believe that all women are slutty.

But you have to understand that most of the women you'll sleep with when you're getting laid off from Tinder and at bars and clubs are going to be freaks. They are the women who can converse with you informally. These places occasionally have good girls, but the majority of the good girls won't be out very often. You'll get to meet a lot of attractive women this way. However, finding a high-quality girl also necessitates looking elsewhere. This is especially true for men who are deciding which girlfriend they want to have children with. Which, as you know, isn't all for you at this time. In addition to traditional places to meet women, the best places to find a potential girlfriend are social circles, conservative neighborhoods, less populated areas, and going out in the world. Institutions of religion Churches, mosques, temples, and other places of worship are examples of religious institutions. Regardless of your culture or what is typical where you live. Religious girls are typically very relationship-focused and sexually conservative. However, the girl you're dating goes out on the weekends even though she attends church or another place once a week. You don't want the woman who rode the cock carousel before converting to religion at the age of thirty. When choosing a girl for a religious organization, look for someone who was involved and active during her prime. You are probably safe if the girl is a religious girl and is 19 years old. Avoid at all costs if she is 30 years old, just had a child, and is switching from a decade of partying to a pious lifestyle. One drawback of dating a lady who practices strict religion is that she could choose to put off having sex until marriage or put it off for a time. To strike a balance, you should look for a female who is open to having sex with men but is picky about who she chooses. This strategy is more long-term and necessitates your spirituality. This is preferable if you want to work hard and are seeking for a female to have children with. It may not be worthwhile if you're younger and only want advice on how to choose your partner for the foreseeable future. *Social networks nightclubs, being available on the market Social networks are another excellent resource for finding the ideal lady. This is so that you can fairly assess a female based on her social network. You may learn more about her history if you two are in the same social circle or if you meet via common connections. You'll be given access to their friends' uncensored tales about other males or her. It's simple to distinguish between females who have been around the block and those who would make excellent pals simply hanging out with them. less populous, traditional places The females are also more suitable for relationships since less populated places tend to be more conservative than cities. Of course, this isn't always the case. However, in general, a girl who hasn't lived in a city and is from a small town or suburb will value relationships more and have a lower-notch count. She also envisions her life in her head in a specific way, which is typically in a committed relationship. Additionally, there is more social pressure to find a man and refrain from prostitution because women in smaller towns tend to settle down earlier. The opposite of what I suggest for all of you who want to be players is living in less populated areas. because having a team and dating multiple women are so ideal in cities. And meeting lots of new women is simple in a city. And I believe you should continue to reside in a city if you are a young man under 30. finding a rural or suburban girl But if you choose a woman from a nearby suburb, you can achieve a happy medium in terms of selecting the right woman. She will still be from a small town that is nearby your city. Girls who are raised close to a city either want nothing to do with it or have aspirations to live there. Finding a girl who is willing to visit you in the city but who does not see herself as a city girl is an important part of learning how to choose the right girlfriend. Although they have a much higher likelihood of going on the cock carousel, you can still date city women. Finding a lady from a city who doesn't have fantasies about it, or one who is from a city but doesn't desire to be there, is preferable. The worst candidates for girlfriends wind up being the females from small villages who have always longed to relocate to the big metropolis. Females who are raised in cities don't have the same fantasies about the sex scene there, and girls who aren't from cities certainly don't care either way. You can always find a beautiful girl in your local area. You guys are aware that I dislike attempting to cold approach every lady I see and playing day games. To get ladies to choose you, I educate you to increase your sexual market worth as much as you can. You may then approach females once they have looked you over. They'll automatically treat you better since they're interested in you.

In actuality, a good girl is always out there waiting to be met. You guys are aware that I dislike trying to cold approach every girl I see and playing day games. To get girls to pick you, I teach you to increase your sexual market value as much as you can. You can then approach girls after they have looked you over. They'll naturally treat you better because they're interested in you. Lift weights, look your best, and walk with utmost assurance. Then you may approach females who are checking you out in public places like the grocery store, the street, the beach, or anywhere else. You participate in life. You don't have time to spend your whole Saturday day meeting women. Keep it till after dark. However, you should remain open to the possibility of meeting a superior female in person when the chance arises. Maintain a good standard of living and approach ladies who make eye contact with you. There are some excellent ladies in the city, but they are often not on Tinder or out at a bar. Of course, we utilize such techniques to meet females. But life circumstances are the finest factor to consider when deciding how to choose your partner. And if you achieve high value in life and become aware of the ladies who are checking you out, situations arise that make it possible for you to meet women. Simply go up to them and start a conversation. Compared to merely cold approaching, you'll chat with a lot fewer ladies. However, since the females you chat to already like you, you'll have far more success with them. signs that your girlfriend wasn't the right one. A woman is dominant in a relationship. Red flags that she isn't as wonderful as you believe will appear after you start dating her And when you've figured out how to choose your partner, you still need to keep an eye on what she does. Because now is the moment to pay attention if you didn't screen thoroughly or if you missed any previous warning signs. Red flags will be covered in a different article. The primary warning indicators that your girlfriend isn't as fantastic as you believe are: Her mother, sisters, and aunts are lewd excessive drinking or partying plenty of buddies that are straight men lived alone in a big city and acknowledged going through a "hoe period" Hasn't decided if she wants to have a family or have children (this will change for 90% of women, but a young woman who doesn't desire this suggests she still wants to ride the cock carousel). has been unmarried for a long time. Choose a good girlfriend pair and a good girlfriend. In the present world, finding a good girlfriend is difficult. However, it's not nearly as bleak as many guys portray it to be online. Yes, there are many ladies with notch counts of 20 to 30 or more males. There are many ladies, nevertheless, who have low notch counts. Since not all women have the potential to be huge sluts. There are a few males who often get laid, but even in that case, it is sufficient to support every lady having a large number of notch counts. This does not imply that females with a notch count of 5 or fewer are perfect. But it's a terrific place to start. Then you may narrow it down to women who are feminine, appreciate relationships, and have the other characteristics you're looking for in a partner. You may find a respectable woman who likes you, too. And you can go down that road if she matches your standards for a top-notch relationship. Not all partnerships will last. In reality, one of you will die or you two will end up splitting up. But how well you pick a girlfriend can greatly influence how much you'll benefit from and enjoy the relationship. Choose the ideal woman, take charge of the relationship, and make the most of it for as long as it contributes to your happiness. Turn into a rebel! follow suit. This prevents a romance from reaching its full potential. However, a really powerful guy who sincerely loves women offers both. He loves and protects his daughter and gives her a sense of security, but he is not paralyzed by worry about losing her. He just needs himself. When there is conflict, he maintains his composure and thinks of ways to make her happy since he already has all he needs. He will open up, admitting his own vulnerabilities as if to say, "Yes, I am broken, too," when she feels exposed by her insecurities or anything going on in her life. It's ok, however. I'm content. He will hug her tight and say just what she wants to hear—nothing—when she needs to weep and feel cherished. Although he cares, he does not cling. Her romantic rock, he is. Never attempt to manipulate a woman. You're doomed to failure. And yet, there are a lot of men who start dating. They insist on her making a pledge to exclusively be with him. I'm sorry, dude. Do not attempt to pass this off as love because it is not. It is not even close to love to want to keep her for yourself. Pure possessiveness, that is. Women are aware of it. They constantly complain to me about how males try to fit them into categories and labels, often with a hint of dissatisfaction or even disdain. Although they dislike the possessiveness, they put up with it because they like the man, therefore "Why not be his girlfriend?" is a reasonable question. But consider this: do you want a lady to stay with you out of a simple "why not"? Do you want her to run into your arms and declare that you are the only person she can think of?

follow suit. This prevents a romance from reaching its full potential. However, a genuinely powerful man who genuinely loves women offers both. He loves and protects his daughter and gives her a sense of security, but he is not paralyzed by worry over losing her. He only needs himself. When there is conflict, he maintains his composure and thinks of ways to make her happy because he already has everything he needs. He will open up, admitting his insecurities as if to say, "Yes, I am broken, too," when she feels exposed by her insecurities or something going on in her life. It's ok, though. I'm content. He will hold her close and say exactly what she needs to hear—nothing—when she needs to cry and feel loved. Although he cares, he does not cling. Her romantic rock, he is. Never attempt to manipulate a woman. You're doomed to failure. And yet, there are a lot of men who start dating. They insist on her pledging to exclusively be with him. I'm sorry, dude. Do not attempt to pass this off as love because it is not. It is not even close to love to want to keep her for yourself. Pure possessiveness, that is. Women are aware of it. They constantly complain to me about how males try to fit them into categories and labels, often with a hint of dissatisfaction or even disdain. Although they dislike the possessiveness, they put up with it because they like the man, therefore "Why not be his girlfriend?" is a reasonable question. But consider this: do you want a lady to stay with you out of a simple "why not"? Do you want her to run into your arms and declare that you are the only person she can think of? Exactly. She wants that as well. You won't need to push for the relationship if the sex is bed-breaking, you two treat one another like royalty, and you adhere to the earlier advice in this article. When she's prepared, she'll let you know. Are you prepared to become her ideal man? That is the only concern you should have right now. Get over your lack of confidence Techniques for Reducing Uncertainty Romanoff offers some coping mechanisms that can make you feel more secure in your bonds with others. Decide what triggers you: Learn to recognize the circumstances that make you feel insecure. Keep a record of the subjects or areas that make you feel insecure so you can start to pinpoint the issues you need to address. Be in touch with your partner: Increase your openness when discussing your insecurities, how they affect your relationship, and how to start overcoming them. Describe your feelings: Try to express your emotions to your partner without pointing the finger at them. Say "I occasionally get stressed because..." instead of "You stress me out because..."

3. Pay attention to your partner: To understand your partner's perspective as well, try to listen to them with an open mind. Use a journal: Maintaining a journal in which you record your thoughts can be beneficial when you're feeling insecure. You can pinpoint situations that make you feel insecure by using the exercise. To assist you and your spouse develop trust, you may even do a couple's activities. Think about seeing a therapist: While awareness and open communication are crucial, there are occasions when you also need the expertise of a professional outsider to help you completely understand how your nervousness is related to more intricate dynamics. Your

therapist may help you deal with your insecurity by working together.

Chapter 4,

Establish a long-lasting, solid connection with her

1. Respect When we respect our spouse, we keep a good opinion of them, which means that our conversations are more likely to build the connection and compassion that are indicators of long-term success. A couple may also hone the ways that they are equal yet distinct using the trait of mutual respect. Respect might lessen the desire to have a superior position in power. Respect may also help someone who has poor self-esteem rise above their predicament.

Respect for one's relationship is important, but respect for oneself is also important. 2. The second attribute required for a strong foundation is friendship. Intimacy, which is the desire to know and be known, is the foundation upon which friendship is built. Like a plant, friendships require maintenance to flourish. When we take care of that fragile place in our hearts where we feel compassion for others, it blossoms. Consider how you might feel if you saw the occasional elderly couple holding hands and grinning as they enter the grocery store. They have found each other through the successes and setbacks of building and sharing a life, and the love that develops from this caring can serve as an example for all of us. The purest desire of our hearts is true friendship. We do not, however, always enjoy our partner. In some cases, we even treat our Beloved worse than a stranger. Because no one can affect us as deeply or as quickly as our partner, we react so heartlessly. They have the power to lead us down into the darkest recesses of our shadow side, far beneath the veneer of civility, politeness, and social graces, to the depths of hatred, rage, and the instinctual urge of "eye for an eye, tooth for a tooth." We have the chance to dcvelop and become more thoughtful about our decisions and less receptive in our actions here, in these shadowy depths. Here, instead of viewing our partner as an adversary or foe, we can decide to foster a friendship. Sometimes it helps to visualize your partner as the Beloved behind the person you're currently disliking in front of you. This quality of friendship requires ongoing attention to detail and deliberate action.

Here are some suggestions to get you going. - Give her what you want.

1. Listening ears, Women sometimes simply need to be heard. Be present, have purposeful dialogues, pay attention to what she has to say, and then give her your thoughts. Make it known that you respect her viewpoints. She will learn two things from this: A) That you value her opinion and your own. B) That you can keep up with her and maybe even help to further her thinking. Bonus points if you surprise her with a gift inspired by a chance encounter. Consider buying her tickets to a performance, a movie, or an exhibition. Even better, take her to her preferred restaurant or get something she expressed like from her favorite retailer.

2. CREATE RELATIONSHIPS WITH PEOPLE WHOM SHE VALUES
   Show a sincere interest in the people she cherishes, whether she is advancing in her career or her family and friends are her life. If she invites you to a professional event, strike up a discussion with her boss and coworkers. If she introduces you to her family members, spend some time getting to know them so that you may later develop a connection with them. It will make her feel good and let her know you care about her.
3. Take action because she wants to. Compromise is a need in relationships even though it may be demanding and keep no one happy. Get out of your comfort zone (and stubbornness) sometimes, and entirely concede to what she wants

simply because she wants it. If you don't like dancing, you may offer to take her out instead, or you could take her on a rare trip to a vineyard where she can have you by her side and weep her eyes out while watching a sad movie. Because she will understand that you are just doing it for her, it will mean much more.

4. BEHAVE AS IF YOU WERE IN A ROM-COM (AT LEAST ONCE)
   Although it might be stressful, buying presents for your girlfriend is rather common. Next time you want to impress your girlfriend, take on a creative project that requires significant thinking, investigation, and effort. Consider writing a collection of poetry for her, making a song about her, beginning a

scrapbook of memories you can add to over time, or making a coupon book where she may exchange tasks, favors, or even sexual acts for you whenever she wants. If she typically prepares meals, take over one evening and establish yourself as the chef of her fantasies. Even if you lack innovation, your effort will get you a "A." (and maybe other things, if you play your cards right). Get going R You shouldn't go out there and attempt to win their favor. To generate interest, you should be pressing the appropriate social buttons. You must learn how to make a girl run after you frantically. I'll give you a few pointers to get her to pursue you. Change how you approach things. Chances are, if you approach a hot woman in a bar, you'll be the 50th guy to do so that hour. Most of those methods would have been the same. Don't follow the herd; do the opposite. You must distinguish yourself from the crowd. Take note of how guys are approaching her and do the complete opposite. Toy with a woman's expectations and break patterns. I've shared a lot of articles about how to develop an effective strategy. Only broken patterns are recognized by the mind. Make her remember you, then move on to engage with other females. The effect of the approach is everything. convey an appealing way of life. Women assess what social security you will offer them as soon as you approach them. It is a typical response to a move. You must demonstrate to them your ability to meet their needs and your exciting way of life, into which she would be happy to step. Sure, your confidence can convey this, but if she's truly interested in you, she'll Google your name and discover all there is to know about you in a matter of seconds. A desirable aura should permeate every aspect of your personal brand. Do not interpret this to mean Lamborghini poses and photos of unnecessary flashiness. You need to project an air of taste and self-confidence. Create a profile on the internet that demonstrates your ability to cover all life's bases. You care about work, home, friends, travel, and recreation. Show that you are a man of values by your actions. Show them a glimpse of the world they would most like to inhabit. The catch is that you have to live that life. Only by visiting new places, collecting stories and photos, going out with friends, and creating lasting memories will you be able to make your life desirable. You may lead the first meeting to offer ladies just the right clue of how wonderful your life is if you work on striking that balance. They'll naturally want to invest since they see themselves as being a part of it.

If you want to know how to get a woman to pursue you, use this advice as well. Perhaps you're just starting to go out and want to keep things a little mysterious by doing something fun without her. Make it a point to keep it a secret until your next encounter, and if she expresses interest in the activity, ask her out to participate in it once again. Showing her that she is a component of your balanced life will add value. appear chosen in advance. It is really attractive to observe a guy who is sought after by other ladies. Other gorgeous ladies want to claim your area right away since you seem to have their approval. The phrase "he only sleeps with models" is one of the nicest things a wingman can utter. He is well-liked by models because they want to bed him! Unconsciously, they believe that by doing the same, they would be placed on an equal footing. It's difficult for a woman to prove herself. Make sure there are pictures of you with lovely ladies online. It will have a comparable impact. Avoid going overboard since it would seem that you are attempting to overcompensate, just as with the Lamborghinis. As you expand your network of gorgeous, bright women, other women will see them in your photos and get curious about the nature of your relationships. Additionally, they'll start seeing any ladies in your photos as rivals. Leave the conclusion unsettled. pique her interest Next, let her pursue you. Disobey the rules. Make the most gorgeous woman in the club wonder why you aren't chatting to her by paying attention to the less attractive ladies there. pique her interest. Increase your social standing in the area but keep her out. She ought to be left wondering why she doesn't know you and why her appearance is ineffective. You're giving off the impression that appearances aren't everything and that your beliefs and interests are diverse. Every time you see one another, keep your emotions and sentiments good. When you see each other, always tip the balance in your favor. You must constantly provide her with a positive, enjoyable experience that makes her feel wonderful. Anchor those good sentiments and make her think of you as having a cozy glow. The strength of connection will be shown by this pattern of positiveness. When your name appears on her phone, she will experience those feelings after you've established a favorable link with your presence. When you see her, always make the interaction more worthwhile. Deepen the discussion by going there. Move forward. Learn about her and share personal information about your life, family, emotions, and experiences. Women speak a language like this. Make use of it often. She will be at ease disclosing this type of information since she will feel as if she has known you for a very long time. Simply put, make her feel good about you and present yourself as a unique person. These are the two main elements that will make her pursue after you. The following are the typical pursuit cues that will pique a woman's interest: When the talk becomes interesting, break off the rapport. Make her want for more. Laugh only when necessary: A good sense of humor may bring people together. You must address the many triggers that women have in various ways. Make her chuckle, then tone down the comedy. pique appetite Suit her: Be aware of the values and characteristics you want in a lady. Don't only limit yourself to the term "hot." She will strive harder to get your attention if she perceives a struggle. Make her wonder why she isn't receiving your attention by using unfavorable body language. Make a little turn away from her to convey that you are uninterested. Develop your reputation as a prize: Make sure it's obvious you're a guy to be wanted, whether you do this by surrounding yourself with attractive ladies, engaging everyone in conversation, or organizing the party itself.

conclusion

in conclusion you must exhibit the traits that a superior woman NEEDS in a guy to win her over and have her pursue after you. Recognize the characteristics that indicate whether a lady will eventually develop into a bitter, LIFE-SUCKING shrew or a dependable source of strength and pleasure. - And a whole lot more

www.ingramcontent.com/pod-product-compliance
Lightning Source LLC
LaVergne TN
LVHW050341160826
845677LV00014B/3732

* 9 7 9 8 3 5 9 0 7 3 5 6 1 *